The Mediterranean Cookbook

25 Quick Recipes to get you started on Cooking the Mediterranean Way!

Copyright © 2015, Lina Sere

All rights Reserved. No part of this publication or the information in it may be quoted from or reproduced in any form by means such as printing, scanning, photocopying or otherwise without prior written permission of the copyright holder.

Disclaimer and Terms of Use:

Effort has been made to ensure that the information in this book is accurate and complete, however, the author and the publisher do not warrant the accuracy of the information, text and graphics contained within the book due to the rapidly changing nature of science, research, known and unknown facts and internet. The Author and the publisher do not hold any responsibility for errors, omissions or contrary interpretation of the subject matter herein. This book is presented solely for motivational and informational purposes only.

Table of Contents

Introduction 5

Breakfast 6

Breakfast Pita Pocket 7

Cheesy Tomato Tart 9

Poppy Lemon Scones 11

Sunflower Seed and Coconut Breakfast Cookies 13

Sweet Raspberry Muesli 15

Lunch 16

Spanish Chicken Costa Brava 17

Cali-Style Fish Tacos 19

Raspberry Couscous Salad 21

Garbanzo and Kidney Bean Salad 23

Fontina Polenta with Mushrooms Sauce 24

Dinner 26

Baked Onion Soup 27

Artichoke and Pesto Pizza 29

Kedgeree 30

Creamy Apricot and Chicken Tajine and 32

Penne and Ricotta Salata 34

Snack 35

Salmon-Stuffed Tomatoes 36

Roasted Grapes and Carrots 38

Spicy Cactus Salsa 39

Fruit and Yogurt Salad 40

Mini Caesar Salads 41

Dessert 42

Avocado Fudge Brownies 43

Salted Caramel and Chocolate Smoothie 45

Squash Bars 46

Banana Peanut Butter Breakfast Casserole 47

Thick PB & B Shake 49

Conclusion 50

Introduction

A majority of the recipes in this book do require you to cook, but many of them are quick and easy so that will be accommodating to your schedule. We've designed them to allow you to spend more time eating and less time cooking. This eBook will definitely take you in the right direction to help you choose the best option for your weight loss. The diets included are Mediterranean Diet-approved, and are here to help you get started on your way to success with eating the Mediterranean way. If you want to live a happier, healthier, life, it starts with your diet and this book is here to help.

While on this diet, you can look to a high amount of legumes, olive oil, unrefined cereals, fruits, and vegetables. While red meat, poultry, and dairy products will be enjoyed in moderation. Hopefully, the information and recipes found in this book will help you get a good grasp on how amazing eating holistic really is. It is my hope to inspire you to incorporate healthy food in your diet every day.

Breakfast

Breakfast Pita Pocket

Yield: Four Servings
Active Time: 20 minutes
Cooking Time: 15 minutes
Total Time: 35 minuets

Ingredients
- 4 whole-grain pita bread pockets
- 1 ½ cup green bell pepper, seeded and chopped
- 2 cups tomatoes, seeded and chopped
- ⅔ cup mild chili peppers, chopped
- 4 garlic cloves, diced
- 4 large free-range eggs, lightly beaten
- 1 tbsp caraway seeds, smashed
- Himalayan Pink salt, to taste
- Freshly ground black pepper, to taste
- 2 tbsp unrefined extra-virgin olive oil (divided)

Method
1. Heat 1 tablespoon olive oil over medium-high heat in a large skillet. Add chili peppers and sauté for a minimum of 5 minutes, or until the peppers become soft. Remove from heat and add to a large bowl.
2. Return the skillet to the stove and heat remaining olive oil. Mix in bell peppers and tomatoes. Sauté for a minimum of 5 minutes, or until the bell peppers become soft. Stir in the eggs, scramble for a minimum of 5 to 10 minutes or until the eggs are set. Stir the egg mixture into the chili pepper mixture. Set to the side.

3. Lightly toast pita bread for a minimum of 1 to 2 minutes on each side in a separate skillet. Evenly divide the egg mixture into four equal servings and place each serving into a pita. Serve immediately.

Cheesy Tomato Tart

Yield: Eight Servings
Active Time: 10 minutes
Cooking Time: 1 hour, 7 minutes
Total Time: 1 hour, 17 minutes

Ingredients
- 2 tomatoes, thinly sliced
- 2 large free-range eggs
- 1 cup whole-wheat bread crumbs
- 1 cup whole-wheat flour
- ½ cup mozzarella cheese, grated
- 1 cup low-fat ricotta
- 1 cup fresh basil, finely chopped
- ½ cup unrefined extra-virgin olive oil
- Cooking spray

Method
1. Set oven to 350 degrees, and coat 9" to 10" tart pan with cooking spray. Set to the side.
2. Combine bread crumbs, flour, and olive oil in a food processor. Blend until dough comes together. Place in the oven to bake for a minimum of 10 to 12 minutes, or until the crust is golden brown.
3. In the meantime, add eggs, ricotta, basil, and mozzarella to a large food processor. Blend until the ingredients are well combined. Set to the side.
4. Place sliced tomatoes on a paper towel and press out excess liquid.
5. Remove tart crust from oven and arrange one layer of tomato slices on the bottom, and top

with cheese mixture. Top with tomato slices and sprinkle with olive oil.
6. Place in the oven to bake for a minimum of 45 to 55 minutes, or until tart is set. Allow tart to cool before serving.

Poppy Lemon Scones

Yield: Twelve Servings
Active Time: 10 minutes
Cooking Time: 15 minutes
Total Time: 25 minutes

Ingredients
- 2 tbsp poppy seeds
- 2 cups unbleached all-purpose flour
- 2 tbsp lemon juice, freshly squeezed
- 2 tbsp lemon peel, grated
- ¾ cup 100% pure cane sugar
- ½ cup full-fat coconut milk
- ½ cup water
- 4 tsp baking powder
- ½ tsp Himalayan Pink salt
- ¾ cup clarified butter

Method
1. Set oven to 400 degrees, and lightly grease a large baking sheet with 1 tablespoon coconut oil. Set to the side.
2. In a large bowl, mix together flour, sugar, salt, and baking powder. Mix well until the ingredients are well combined. Cut in the butter until the mixture is finely coarse. Slowly stir in poppy seeds, lemon zest, coconut milk, and lemon juice. Stir until the mixture becomes smooth and thick.
3. Add even portions of the batter onto the prepared baking sheet about 3" apart.
4. Place in the oven to bake for a minimum of 10 to 15 minutes or until the scones are well done

and golden brown. Remove from the oven and allow to cool before serving.

Sunflower Seed and Coconut Breakfast Cookies

Yield: Twelve Servings
Active Time: 10 minutes
Cooking Time: 12 minutes
Total Time: 22 minutes

Ingredients
- ½ cup sunflower seeds
- 1 ¼ cup quick-cooking rolled oats
- 1 cup whole-wheat pastry flour
- ½ cup unsweetened coconut, grated
- 1 large free-range egg
- ¾ tsp baking powder
- ½ cup monk fruit sweetener
- 2 tsp vanilla extract
- ½ cup unrefined virgin coconut oil

Method
1. Set oven to 375 degrees, and line two large baking sheets with parchment paper.
2. Beat together coconut oil, sweetener, egg, and vanilla in a medium bowl using an electric mixer.
3. Fold in the grated coconut and sunflowers seeds. Set to side.
4. In a large bowl, combine oats, baking powder, and flour, mix well to blend ingredients. Make a well in the center of the bowl. Add egg mixture to the well, and stir until dough is thoroughly blended.
5. Place rounded tablespoons of the dough onto the lined baking sheets. Be sure the each

portion of dough are well separated to prevent dough cookies from baking together.
6. Place in the oven to bake for a minimum of 10 to 12 minutes, or until cookies are lightly browned. Serve immediately.

Sweet Raspberry Muesli

Yield: Five Servings
Active Time: 10 minutes
Chill Time: 2 hours
Total Time: 2 hours, 10 minutes

Ingredients
- 1 cup rolled-oats
- ¼ cup oat bran
- 1 cup fresh raspberries
- 3 tbsp dried apricots, chopped
- 3 tbsp dried figs, chopped
- 3 tbsp pitted dates, chopped
- ½ cup toasted walnuts, coarsely chopped
- 1 cup plain low-fat yogurt
- 1 cup low-fat milk
- ⅓ cup organic raw honey

Method
1. In a large mixing bowl, mix together oats, oat bran, yogurt, milk, walnuts, honey, and dried fruits.
2. Cover with plastic wrap and place oat mixture in the fridge to chill for a minimum of 2 hours.
3. When ready to serve, top each serving with an even portion of raspberries. Serve immediately.

Lunch

Spanish Chicken Costa Brava

Yield: Four Servings
Active Time: 15 minutes
Cooking Time: 20 minutes
Total Time: 35 minutes

Ingredients
- 10 boneless, skinless chicken breasts, cut in half
- 1 large red bell pepper, thinly sliced
- 1 large yellow onion, quartered
- 2 garlic cloves, minced
- 2 ½ cup pineapple chunks, juice drained and reserved
- 1 (14.5 ounce) can stewed tomatoes
- 2 cups black olives
- 2 tbsp organic cornstarch
- 2 tbsp water
- ½ cup spicy salsa
- 1 tsp ground cumin
- 1 tsp ground cinnamon
- Himalayan Pink salt, to taste
- Freshly ground black pepper, to taste
- 1 tbsp unrefined extra-virgin olive oil

Method
1. Add pineapples to a large bowl and season with salt. Set to the side.
2. Heat olive oil in a large skillet over medium-high heat. Add the chicken halves. Sear the chicken halves for a minimum of 2 minutes on each side, or until each side is browned.

3. Add the garlic and onion and sauté for an additional 2 to 3 minutes or until the onions become soft. Season with cumin and cinnamon.
4. Stir in the reserved pineapple juice, tomatoes, olives, and salsa. Cover and cook for a minimum of 25 minutes.
5. In a small bowl, combine cornstarch and water. Mix until the mixture becomes thick and milky. Pour into the chicken mixture.
6. Add bell peppers and bring to a boil. Once the mixture thickens add pineapples. Remove from heat. Serve immediately.

Cali-Style Fish Tacos

Yield: Four Servings
Active Time: 15 minutes
Cooking Time: 20 minutes
Total Time: 35 minutes

Ingredients
- 3 wild-caught mahi mahi fillets
- 8 (6 inch) yellow corn tortillas
- 1 ripe avocado, peeled, cored, and cut into wedges
- 2 cups green cabbage, thinly sliced
- 2 scallions, finely chopped
- ½ cup red onion, finely chopped
- 1 tbsp lime juice, freshly squeezed
- ¾ tsp coriander powder
- ¾ tsp chili powder
- ¼ tsp Himalayan Pink salt
- Freshly ground black pepper
- 2 tsp unrefined extra-virgin olive oil
- Cooking spray

Method
1. Set oven to 350 degrees and coat a 7"x11" baking dish with cooking spray. Set to the side.
2. In a small bowl, combine lime juice, olive oil, coriander, chili powder, and salt. Mix well until the ingredients are emulsified. Brush the fish with the lime juice mixture on both sides, and place into the prepared baking dish.
3. Place the fish in the oven to bake for a minimum of 15 to 20 minutes or until fish is

easily flaked with a fork. Remove from oven, flake the fish, and set to the side to cool.
4. In a medium bowl, mix together scallion, onion, cabbage, salt, and pepper.
5. Place each tortilla onto a flat surface and top with 2 tablespoons of the cabbage mixture, 2 tablespoons of the mahi mahi, and top off with an additional tablespoon of the cabbage mixture. Fold tortillas in half to form a taco.
6. Serve each taco with one slice of avocado. Garnish each with an additional squeeze of lime juice if desired.

Raspberry Couscous Salad

Yield: Six Servings
Active Time: 10 minutes
Cooking Time: 10 minutes
Total Time: 20 minutes

Ingredients
- 1 ½ cup golden couscous
- 2 large zucchinis, thinly sliced
- 4 green onions, sliced diagonally
- ⅓ cup toasted pine nuts
- 1 ½ cup fresh raspberries
- 2 cups low-sodium chicken stock
- 1 ½ cup feta cheese, crumbled
- 1 tbsp white wine vinegar
- 1 tbsp balsamic vinegar
- 2 tbsp lemon juice, freshly squeezed
- ¼ cup fresh basil, finely chopped
- Himalayan Pink salt, to taste
- Freshly ground black pepper, to taste
- ¼ cup unrefined extra-virgin olive oil

Method
1. Add chicken stock to a boil in a large saucepan and slowly stir in the couscous. Remove from heat and cover with lid. Allow the couscous to sit for a minimum of 10 minutes, or until the chicken stock is fully absorbed.
2. In a medium bowl, mix together olive oil, lemon juice, white wine vinegar, balsamic vinegar, salt, and pepper. Mix well until the ingredients are emulsified. Set to the side.

3. Add the couscous and remaining ingredients to a large salad bowl. Stir to evenly distribute the ingredients. Pour the olive oil mixture over the salad. Toss well to coat. Serve immediately.

Garbanzo and Kidney Bean Salad

Yield: Four Servings
Active Time: 20 minutes
Chill Time: 2 hours
Total Time: 2 hours, 20 minutes

Ingredients
- 2 cups cooked garbanzo beans
- 2 cups cooked kidney beans
- 1 medium tomato, chopped
- ½ cup red onion, finely chopped
- 2 tbsp fresh lemon juice, freshly squeezed
- 1 tbsp lemon zest, freshly grated
- ½ cup fresh parsley, finely chopped
- 1 tsp capers, rinsed and drained
- Himalayan Pink salt, to taste
- Freshly ground black pepper, to taste
- 3 tbsp unrefined extra-virgin olive oil

Method
1. Mix all of the ingredients together in a large salad bowl. Stir thoroughly to evenly distribute ingredients. Cover the bowl with plastic wrap.
2. Place the bowl in the fridge to chill for a minimum of 2 hours before serving.

Fontina Polenta with Mushrooms Sauce

Yield: Four Servings
Active Time: 5 minutes
Cooking Time: 15 minutes
Total Time: 20 minutes

Ingredients
- 8 ounces cremini mushrooms
- 8 ounces exotic mushroom blend, chopped
- ¾ cup instant polenta
- 3 garlic cloves, minced
- 2 cups organic vegetable broth (divided)
- 2 cups full-fat coconut milk
- 1 cup Fontina cheese, shredded (divided)
- 2 tsp lemon juice, freshly squeezed
- 1 tsp fresh thyme, finely chopped
- Himalayan Pink salt, to taste
- Freshly ground black pepper, to taste
- 2 tbsp unrefined extra-virgin olive oil

Method
1. In a large skillet, heat olive oil over high heat. Toss in the mushrooms and sauté for a minimum of 5 minutes. Add garlic and thyme. Sauté for an additional 60 seconds. Slowly stir in about ⅓ cup broth, lemon juice, salt, and pepper.
2. In a medium saucepan, bring milk and remaining broth to a boil. Slowly stir in polenta and allow to cook for a minimum of 5 minutes or until the polenta has absorbed the liquid.

3. Stirring constantly, add the cheese and salt as desired. Stir until the cheese is melted. Remove from heat.
4. When ready to serve top each serving with the mushroom mixture and enjoy!

Dinner

Baked Onion Soup

Yield: Eight Servings
Active Time: 15 minutes
Cooking Time: 45 minutes
Total Time: 1 hour

Ingredients
- 1 pound yellow onions, thinly sliced
- 1 pound red onions, thinly sliced
- 2 cups green onions, finely chopped
- 16 slices baguette, cut into 3" rounds
- 2 ½ cups beef stock
- 2 ½ cups chicken stock
- 4 tbsp sour cream
- 1 ½ cup Parmesan cheese
- ¾ pound Gruyère cheese, grated
- ½ stick grass-fed butter
- Unrefined extra-virgin olive oil

Method
1. Set oven to 425 degrees, and lightly grease a large casserole dish with olive oil. Set to the side.
2. In a large saucepan, melt butter over medium-high heat. Toss in the onions and sauté for a minimum of 5 to 10 minutes or until the onions are tender and slightly browned.
3. Slowly stir in the chicken stock and salt. Bring to a boil and allow to simmer for a minimum of 15 minutes and stir in sour cream. Remove from heat and set to the side.
4. Coat each slice of baguette with olive oil on both sides, and half of the bread in the bottom of the prepared casserole dish. Season each

slice with salt and pepper and top with half of the Gruyère cheese.
5. Add the final layer of bread and season with salt and pepper and a final layer of Gruyère cheese. Top with a single layer of green onions and Parmesan cheese. Pour onion mixture over the top.
6. Place in the oven to bake for a minimum of 15 to 20 minutes or until the soup is bubbly and slightly browned. Serve immediately.

Artichoke and Pesto Pizza

Yield: Four Servings
Active Time: 10 minutes
Cooking Time: 12 minutes
Total Time: 22 minutes

Ingredients
- 1 large whole-wheat pizza crust
- ½ cup artichoke hearts, drained and pulled apart
- 3 Roma tomatoes, thinly sliced
- 2 tbsp Kalamata olives
- 2 tbsp hot chili peppers
- 1 (4 ounce) jar organic basil pesto
- 2 tbsp unbleached all-purpose flour
- ⅓ cup feta cheese, crumbled
- Cooking spray

Method
1. Set oven to 450 degrees, and lightly coat a large, flat pizza pan with cooking spray. Set to the side.
2. Lightly flour your working surface with the flour. Place the pizza crust onto the surface. Spread the pesto sauce over the pizza crust.
3. Arrange the tomatoes, artichokes, olives, and hot chili pepper over the pizza. Sprinkle the feta cheese over the top.
4. Transfer the pizza to the prepared pizza pan. Place in the oven to bake for a minimum of 10 to 12 minutes, or until the crust is crisp and the feta cheese has melted. Cut into slices and serve immediately.

Kedgeree

Yield: Two Servings
Active Time: 20 minutes
Cooking Time: 32 minutes
Total Time: 52 minutes

Ingredients
- 4 ounces smoked Mahi Mahi
- 2 cups uncooked basmati rice
- ¼ cup frozen green peas
- 4 green onions, finely chopped
- 4 large eggs
- 1 cup full-fat coconut milk
- ½ cup plain Greek yogurt
- 1 bay leaf
- Himalayan Pink salt, to taste
- Freshly ground black pepper, to taste
- 1 tbsp clarified butter

Method
1. Cook the rice according to the package instructions. Drain and set to the side.
2. In a large saucepan, bring the eggs to a boil over medium-high heat. Immediately remove the saucepan from the heat, cover, and allow the eggs to stand in the hot water for a minimum of 10 to 12 minutes. When ready, peel and chop the eggs. Set to the side.
3. Add the Mahimahi to a small skillet and pour in the coconut milk. Be sure that the fish is fully submerged in the coconut milk. Add the bay leaf and bring to a boil over medium heat. Allow the fish to cook for a minimum of 5 to 10 minutes or until the fish is easily flaked with a

fork. Remove from heat, drain, and discard the bay leaf. Flake the fish and set to the side.
4. Melt butter in a large skillet over medium-high heat and slowly stir in the curry powder. Add the peas and green onions. Sauté for a minimum of 5 minutes or until the vegetables become tender.
5. Mix in the chopped eggs, cooked rice, flaked fish, salt and pepper. Stir until the ingredients are evenly distributed. Cook for about 5 minutes. Remove from heat and serve immediately with yogurt.

Creamy Apricot and Chicken Tajine and

Yield: Four Servings
Active Time: 5 minutes
Cooking Time: 1 hour, 33 minutes
Total Time: 3 hours, 38 minutes

Ingredients
- 8 chicken thighs, skin removed
- 8 dried apricots
- 2 large onions, finely chopped
- 2 garlic clove, minced
- 1 fennel bulb, chopped
- ½ cup raisins
- ¾ cup heavy cream
- 6 ounces Gouda cheese, shredded
- 2 tbsp fresh parsley, finely chopped
- 2 tbsp fresh thyme, finely chopped
- 2 tbsp fresh cilantro, finely chopped
- 1 tsp coriander
- 1 tsp cumin
- 1 tsp turmeric
- 1 tsp paprika
- 1 tsp dried ginger
- 3 cups coconut water
- Unrefined virgin coconut oil, melted
- Himalayan Pink salt, to taste
- Freshly ground black pepper, to taste

Method
1. Cut a slit into each of the chicken thighs, and place each thigh into a large bowl along with 3 tablespoon garlic, coconut oil, parsley, thyme, coriander, cumin, turmeric, paprika, and ginger.

Mix well to combine. Cover and place in the fridge to marinate and chill for a minimum of 2 hours.
2. When chicken is ready, heat 2 tablespoons of coconut oil and chicken in a large skillet. Cook the chicken for 3 minutes on each side, or until the chicken is browned on each sides. Add onions, fennel, coconut water, heavy cream, cheese, apricots, cilantro, raisins, salt, and pepper.
3. Cover up chicken and allow to cook for a minimum of 1 ½ hours.

Penne and Ricotta Salata

Yield: Eight Servings
Active Time: 5 minutes
Cooking Time: 1 hour, 33 minutes
Total Time: 1 hour, 20 minutes

Ingredients
- 10 ounces uncooked whole-grain penne pasta
- 4 pounds yellow onions, thinly sliced
- 2 cups toasted walnuts, crushed
- 1 pound ricotta salata, crumbled
- 1 ½ tbsp lemon juice, freshly squeezed
- ⅔ cup fresh parsley, finely chopped
- 1 tsp 100% pure cane sugar
- Himalayan Pink salt, to taste
- Freshly ground black pepper, to taste
- 5 tbsp unrefined extra-virgin olive oil (divided)

Method
1. Heat 3 tablespoons olive oil over high heat in a large skillet. Stir in onions, sugar, and salt. Sauté until the onions become tender and golden, or for a minimum of 5 to 10 minutes.
2. Reduce the heat to medium and simmer for a minimum of 35 to 40 minutes. Stir occasionally. Remove from heat.
3. In the meantime, bring the penne pasta to a boil. Simmer for a minimum of 9 to 12 minutes. Remove from heat and drain. Reserve ½ cup of the cooking liquid.
4. Add the pasta to a large bowl. Stir in the parsley, walnuts, ricotta salata, cooking liquid, lemon juice, salt, pepper, and remaining olive oil. Serve immediately.

Snack

Salmon-Stuffed Tomatoes

Yield: Four Servings
Active Time: 20 minutes
Cooking Time: 8 minutes
Total Time: 28 minutes

Ingredients
- 4 medium tomatoes, halved and seeds and pulp removed
- 8 ounces smoked Salmon, coarsely chopped
- 4 tbsp cream cheese
- 4 tbsp goat cheese, crumbled
- 2 tsp Parmesan cheese, grated
- 10 free-range eggs, lightly beaten
- 2 tbsp heavy cream
- ¼ cup fresh chives, finely chopped
- ½ tbsp fresh rosemary, finely chopped
- ½ tbsp fresh summer savory, finely chopped
- 1 tbsp fresh parsley, finely chopped
- 2 tbsp unrefined extra-virgin olive oil (More if needed)

Method
1. Set oven to broil. Line a large baking sheet with aluminum foil, and arrange tomato halves onto the prepared baking sheet. Set to the side.
2. In a medium bowl, mix together rosemary, summer savory, and parsley. Mix well until the ingredients are thoroughly combined. Set to the side.
3. Using 1 tablespoon olive oil, brush the inside and outside of each tomato half and season with the herb mixture. Place the tomatoes into

the oven to broil for a minimum of 3 minutes. Immediately turn off the broiler, and leave the tomatoes in the oven.
4. In a large skillet, heat the remaining olive oil over medium heat. Add eggs, heavy cream, smoked salmon, cream cheese, goat cheese, and chives. Using a fork, scramble the egg mixture until the eggs are set, or for a minimum of 5 minutes.
5. Remove the tomato halves from the oven and stuff each with about ¼ cup of the salmon mixture. Top each stuffed tomato with Parmesan cheese. Serve immediately.

Roasted Grapes and Carrots

Yield: Six Servings
Active Time: 15 minutes
Cooking Time: 20 minutes
Total Time: 35 minutes

Ingredients
- 1 pound baby carrots
- 2 pounds red seedless grapes
- 1 medium red onion, cut into wedges
- 1 tsp ground cumin
- 2 tbsp unrefined extra-virgin olive oil

Method
1. Set oven to 375 degrees, and line a large baking sheet with aluminum foil. Set to the side.
2. In a large bowl, add carrots, grapes, onion, and olive oil. Toss well to coat. Season with cumin and mix well to combine.
3. Dump the carrot mixture onto the prepared baking sheet and spread out into an even layer.
4. Place in the oven to roast for a minimum of 15 to 20 minutes.

Spicy Cactus Salsa

Yield: Four Servings
Active Time: 5 minutes
Chill Time: 2 hours
Total Time: 2 hours, 5 minutes

Ingredients
- 1 cup cactus, rinsed and roughly chopped
- 3 large tomatoes, finely chopped
- 2 ripe avocados, peeled and chopped
- ¼ red onion, finely chopped
- 1 jalapeño, seeded and finely chopped
- ¼ cup fresh cilantro, finely chopped
- 2 tbsp lime juice, freshly squeezed
- Himalayan Pink salt, to taste
- Freshly ground black pepper, to taste

Method
1. In a large bowl, combine all of the ingredients. Mix well to combine.
2. Pour the ingredients into a serving bowl and cover with plastic wrap. Place the bowl in the fridge to chill for a minimum of 2 hours.
3. When ready to serve, enjoy with favorite chip or vegetable.

Fruit and Yogurt Salad

Yield: Six Servings
Active Time: 10 minutes
Chill Time: 2 hours
Total Time: 2 hours, 10 minutes

Ingredients
- 1 large cup bananas, sliced
- 1 cup fresh strawberries, leaves removed and sliced
- 2 cups organic green apples, chopped
- 1 cup roasted walnuts, roughly chopped
- 1 ½ cup plain Greek yogurt
- 1 tsp ground cinnamon

Method
1. In a large bowl, combine all ingredients by slowly folding them into the yogurt. Place the ingredients into a large serving bowl and cover with plastic wrap.
2. Place the salad in the fridge to chill for about 1 to 2 hours before serving.

Mini Caesar Salads

Yield: Sixteen Servings
Active Time: 15 minutes
Cooking Time: 5 minutes
Total Time: 20 minutes

Ingredients
- 2 boneless, skinless, grilled chicken breasts, shredded
- 8 (8") whole-wheat tortillas
- ½ cup romaine lettuce, finely chopped
- ¼ cup whole kernel corn, cooked
- ⅜ cup Parmesan cheese, grated (divided)
- 4 grape tomatoes, quartered
- 3 tbsp Caesar dressing
- Cooking spray

Method
1. Set oven to 375 degrees, and lightly coat a 16-cup mini muffin pan with cooking spray. Sprinkle 2 tablespoon Parmesan cheese onto the sides and bottoms of each muffin cup. Set to the side.
2. Cut out 16 (2 ½") rounds from each tortilla. Place each round into each muffin cup.
3. Place in the oven to bake for a minimum of 5 minutes. Remove from oven and allow to cool.
4. In a medium bowl, stir together chicken and Caesar dressing. Set aside.
5. Add an even portion of lettuce, chicken, corn, and tomatoes to each tortilla cup. Sprinkle with remaining cheese. Serve immediately.

Dessert

Avocado Fudge Brownies

Yield: Eight Servings
Active Time: 10 minutes
Cooking Time: 22 minutes
Total Time: 32 minutes

Ingredients
- ⅓ cup avocado, mashed
- ¼ cup toasted walnuts, chopped
- ¾ cup cocoa powder
- ⅓ cup chocolate chips
- ⅔ cup whole-wheat pastry flour
- 1 tbsp tapioca starch
- ⅓ cup Grade A maple syrup
- ¼ cup almond milk
- ¾ cup 100% pure cane sugar
- 2 tsp vanilla extract
- ½ tsp baking powder
- ½ tsp baking soda
- ¼ Himalayan Pink salt
- ¼ cup unrefined extra-virgin coconut oil, melted

Method
1. Set oven to 350 degrees and line an 8"x8" baking dish with parchment paper. Set to the side.
2. In a large food processor, blend avocado, coconut oil, sugar, syrup, vanilla extract, and milk. Blend until a smooth and creamy consistency is reached. Set to the side.

3. Combine cocoa powder, starch, baking powder, baking soda, and salt in a large bowl. Mix well to combine and form a well in the center. Pour the avocado mixture into the well and mix well to blend. Add the chocolate chips and walnuts, and transfer the mixture into the lined baking dish.
4. Place in the oven to bake for a minimum of 20 to 22 minutes or until the brownies are well-done but moist.
5. Remove from oven and allow to cool for a minimum of 15 minutes before serving.

Salted Caramel and Chocolate Smoothie

Yield: Two Servings
Active Time: 5 minutes
Blending Time: 5 minutes
Total Time: 10 minutes

Ingredients
- 2 tbsp organic salted caramel
- 1 tbsp cacao powder
- 2 tbsp cacao nibs
- 2 cups organic coconut ice cream
- 1 cup full-fat coconut milk
- 2 large bananas, halved
- 1 tsp vanilla bean powder

Method
1. In a large blender, add the caramel, milk, cacao nibs, and ice cream. Blend at medium to high speed for a minimum of 2 to 3 minutes, or until a smooth consistency is reached.
2. Add the cacao powder, vanilla bean powder, and bananas to the blender and blend for an additional 2 to 3 minutes or until the mixture becomes smooth.
3. Pour into two separate serving glasses or enjoy one large serving by yourself!

Squash Bars

Yield: Twelve Servings
Active Time: 15 minutes
Cooking Time: 45 minutes
Total Time: 1 hour

Ingredients
- 2 cups butternut squash, pureed
- 8 large eggs, separated
- 1 tbsp ground cinnamon
- 2 tbsp unrefined virgin coconut oil

Method
1. Set oven to 350 degrees, and line a 9"x13" baking dish with parchment paper. Set to the side.
2. Using a whisk, beat together egg whites in a large bowl until the egg whites become fluffy. Set to the side.
3. In a separate bowl, mix together egg yolks, squash, cinnamon, and coconut oil. Mix well until the ingredients are well blended. Gently fold in the egg whites and pour into the prepared baking dish.
4. Place in the oven to bake for a minimum of 40 to 45 minutes, or until eggs are set. Remove from the oven and allow to cool.
5. When ready to serve, cut into twelve bars. Store the remainder in an airtight container and place in the fridge.

Banana Peanut Butter Breakfast Casserole

Yield: Sixteen Servings
Active Time: 20 minutes
Cooking Time: 55 minutes
Total Time: 1 hour, 15 minutes

Ingredients
- 2 cans organic honey butter biscuits, chilled
- 1 cup organic creamy peanut butter
- 4 large bananas, sliced
- 6 large eggs, lightly beaten
- 3 cups full-fat coconut milk
- ½ cup monk fruit sweetener
- ½ cup organic raw honey
- 3 tbsp unrefined virgin coconut oil (divided)

Method
1. Set oven to 350 degrees and lightly grease a large baking sheet and 4-quart baking dish with 1 tablespoon coconut oil.
2. Arrange the banana slices onto the bottom of the prepared baking dish in a single layer. Set to the side.
3. Separate biscuits the biscuit dough and arrange the biscuits about 2 inches apart onto the prepared baking dish. Bake the biscuits according the instructions on the packaging. Once the biscuits are ready, remove from the oven and set to the side to cool for a minimum of 10 minutes.
4. In the meantime, add the eggs, sweetener, honey, and coconut milk to a large bowl. Using a whisk, beat the ingredients together until a

smooth consistency is reached. Set to the side.
5. Once the biscuits are cool enough to handle, slice the biscuits in half and spread an even amount of peanut butter on the bottom half of each biscuit, and cover with the top half. Add the biscuit sandwiches to the egg mixture and allow them to soak for a minimum of 5 minutes.
6. When ready, add each of the soaked sandwiches into the banana-lined baking dish by arranging them carefully on top of the banana slices.
7. Place in oven and bake for a minimum of 35 to 40 minutes, or until the casserole is golden brown. Remove from oven and allow to cool before serving.

Banana Peanut Butter Breakfast Casserole

Yield: Sixteen Servings
Active Time: 20 minutes
Cooking Time: 55 minutes
Total Time: 1 hour, 15 minutes

Ingredients
- 2 cans organic honey butter biscuits, chilled
- 1 cup organic creamy peanut butter
- 4 large bananas, sliced
- 6 large eggs, lightly beaten
- 3 cups full-fat coconut milk
- ½ cup monk fruit sweetener
- ½ cup organic raw honey
- 3 tbsp unrefined virgin coconut oil (divided)

Method
1. Set oven to 350 degrees and lightly grease a large baking sheet and 4-quart baking dish with 1 tablespoon coconut oil.
2. Arrange the banana slices onto the bottom of the prepared baking dish in a single layer. Set to the side.
3. Separate biscuits the biscuit dough and arrange the biscuits about 2 inches apart onto the prepared baking dish. Bake the biscuits according the instructions on the packaging. Once the biscuits are ready, remove from the oven and set to the side to cool for a minimum of 10 minutes.
4. In the meantime, add the eggs, sweetener, honey, and coconut milk to a large bowl. Using a whisk, beat the ingredients together until a

smooth consistency is reached. Set to the side.
5. Once the biscuits are cool enough to handle, slice the biscuits in half and spread an even amount of peanut butter on the bottom half of each biscuit, and cover with the top half. Add the biscuit sandwiches to the egg mixture and allow them to soak for a minimum of 5 minutes.
6. When ready, add each of the soaked sandwiches into the banana-lined baking dish by arranging them carefully on top of the banana slices.
7. Place in oven and bake for a minimum of 35 to 40 minutes, or until the casserole is golden brown. Remove from oven and allow to cool before serving.

Thick PB & B Shake

Yield: Four Servings
Active Time: 10 minutes
Blending Time: 7 minutes
Freezing Time: 2 hours
Total Time: 2 hours, 17 minutes

Ingredients
- 8 slightly ripe bananas, cut into chunks
- ¾ cup organic, natural peanut butter
- 4 to 15 drops Stevia extract
- 1 cup full-fat coconut milk or desired amount
- 4 drops vanilla extract

Method
1. Place banana chunks on a medium serving plate, and place in freezer. Allow bananas to freeze for a minimum of 2 hours or until the banana chunks become solid.
2. In a food processor or blender, process the frozen bananas, Stevia, coconut milk, and vanilla extract for a minimum of 5 to 7 minutes, or until the mixture becomes smooth and creamy.
3. Discontinue blending and add peanut butter. Restart the blending until peanut butter is well incorporated and mixture is smooth. Serve immediately and enjoy!

Conclusion

It is my hope that you will be successful with the Mediterranean Diet. I want you to stick with eating like you want to be healthy and happy. However, if this is something that you think you will not be able to do for an extended amount of time, that's okay. At least you will become more knowledgeable of the foods that you are eating, and more aware of what to eat and what not to eat. Consider this eBook as an introduction to the world of holistic eating! To achieve the best results, remember to check all food labels. There are a lot of hidden carbs, additives, and sugars hiding in our foods.

Good luck with your diet, and I hope that you will be have great success!

www.ingramcontent.com/pod-product-compliance
Lightning Source LLC
LaVergne TN
LVHW020030030125
800364LV00008B/855